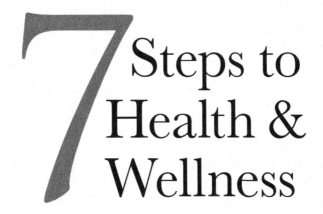
7 Steps to Health & Wellness

Follow these 7 easy steps and experience life - one you have always dreamed of.

Sonja Christiansen, KRMT

Healing Focus

Focused Healing and Kruna Reiki Master Teacher

authorHOUSE®

AuthorHouse™
1663 Liberty Drive
Bloomington, IN 47403
www.authorhouse.com
Phone: 1 (800) 839-8640

© *2016 Sonja Christiansen, KRMT. All rights reserved.*

No part of this book may be reproduced, stored in a retrieval system, or transmitted by any means without the written permission of the author.

Published by AuthorHouse 02/19/2016

ISBN: 978-1-5049-7736-4 (sc)
ISBN: 978-1-5049-7734-0 (hc)
ISBN: 978-1-5049-7735-7 (e)

Library of Congress Control Number: 2016901810

Print information available on the last page.

Any people depicted in stock imagery provided by Thinkstock are models, and such images are being used for illustrative purposes only.
Certain stock imagery © Thinkstock.

This book is printed on acid-free paper.

Because of the dynamic nature of the Internet, any web addresses or links contained in this book may have changed since publication and may no longer be valid. The views expressed in this work are solely those of the author and do not necessarily reflect the views of the publisher, and the publisher hereby disclaims any responsibility for them.

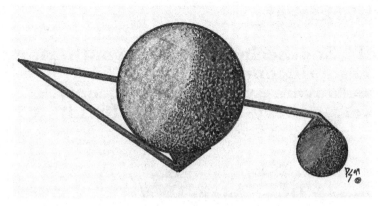

CREDITS

Forward:

Ed Webber

Back Cover Review:

Nathan Harper, MS, APRN-CNP, Board Certified Family Nurse Practitioner

Editing, Organizing and Biography:

Cheri Wheeler, BSN, RN

Medical Consultation:

"Doc" Nathan Harper
Dr. Stanley Painter D.O.

Artwork:

Paul Southerland (paul_southerland@rocketmail.com)
Anna Moyers (www.facebook.com/moyers-gallery-1660306090916243)

Review & Discussion:

Eddie & Karen Owens
Jackie Martin
Jill Stinson
Linda Smith
Pat Hanrahan
Sue Martin
Sylvia Plourde
Teresa Black
Vagina Espansosa
Fuzz

A special thank you to Ali, from the National Qigong Association
For their permission to include their information in this book.

Dedication & Thanks

This is dedicated to my grandfather, Joseph Mulla. He was a Homeopathic Physician during the first and second world wars in Germany. He was a strong believer in fresh air and sunshine, eating properly, chewing your food 23 times for each forkful and outdoor exercise. In those days he was also a surgeon and an herbalist as well as a "Laying on-of Hands" energy healer. Today we call this Homeopathic Energy Medicine.

I want to say thank you to all of my friends and family around the country for their help with all the things I usually need help with. I could not do this without your encouragement, corrections and support. A special thank you to my Little Fuzzy Guy for his non stop support, no matter what.

Foreword

58 years ago I met a little girl named Sonja. She was a barefoot wonder with honey-blond hair and 12 brothers and sisters. She asked many questions and was never quite satisfied with the answers. She spent most of her time caring for her siblings. In those years she learned and studied many old farmers remedies for various ailments that would come along and listened intently to her grandfathers stories. He was a Doctor and a naturalist healer in his own right. She learned about plants and especially the relationships between the poison ones and the ones that healed, such as Poison Ivy, Sweet Grass and Jewel Weed, which are some of the poisons and cures that grow right next to each other. These correlations fascinated her.

In later years, as a teenager and young woman she studied with people who were Spiritualists as well as Native Healers who crossed her path. She never missed a chance to learn from elders.

Here we are 58 years later and she still has that same curiosity. She has traveled to China to study under the Chi Masters and has learned many healing modalities for mind, body, and spirit. She also learned that experience could be a great teacher. Recently she had to have a kidney removed and is using her knowledge to combat the residual effects from the surgery and the medications she has had to take.

Her philosophy is to use all that Spirit has made available to us. The doctors, medicines and therapies provided by "standard" medicine as well as the ancient cures of "Alternative" medicine. As she tells people, "Use all that you have at your disposal, but do so responsibly. Learn what you need, and study each thing as if it meant your life." This is a good policy. Get a read on the track record of each therapy before putting it into use for YOUR body, mind and spirit. Be a working partner with your medical professionals. Let them know you want to be a partner with them in bringing about the best possible results from your healthcare.

This book will lead you to, 1. Understanding your body and it's needs and 2. How to work with your body to get the best from it. Simplicity does not mean simplistic. This book will take you step by step, with explicit instructions. There will be nothing to buy after you have finished. You will be amazed, re-energized and much more calm. Enjoy it and the good health that can simply be yours.

Ed Webber

Lifetime friend and student.

Healers I Have Known.

Over the years I have known a number of people I have considered healers. They have impacted my life in many ways and have brought me to this book today.

Their common denominator was their love and compassion for all people.

Dr. Collins, M.D.

Was my first. He was still birthing babies during home visits in Liberty, Me., when I was twelve. He had a unique knowledge of his communities and the people in them. An "old country doc". who knew what to do to help, regardless which side of the law you might find yourself on.

Dr. Stanley Painter, D.O.

A man who could talk to any of his country patients about anything from rock formations, how to plant a garden, raise violets or which herbs to use for what. He calmed them down so he could get to the heart of things. He was one to always look out for and help the little guy. He was there when you needed him at your house or in his driveway, in Winthrop, Me. waiting for you with the medicine that would save your life in his hands. I know. He saved mine.

Dr. Edith Chitman, Ph.D.

Always knew how to show compassion to others. Whether or not they could pay. She would always help the best she could, in every way she could. She never thought you were nuts because you might see or hear things others didn't. Any one who came to see her always felt safe.

"Doc." Nathan Harper.

A true healer in every sense of the word. Not only through conversation, but also through his research. You can trust him to be part of the solution you needed for your best recovery. His community loves and trusts him. His energy is always positive. He sees his patients through the eye of his heart.

Elka Gebhard

An Herbalist. She came here from Germany after WW2. She was a scientist in her working life. She knew the name of every herb and mushroom that grew in her area in Maine as well as how to find and use them. She knew a great deal about the old remedies before the use of modern medicine. She accepted the ideas and thoughts of modern medicine and found common ground between them. She would offer her knowledge to any one who would ask and was serious. She suffered no fools.

Rev. Abbie Perry

A spiritual hands-on-healer, who understood the interaction between the physical and spiritual plane of thought and vibration. I was blessed to study under her for many years. She was well known throughout the United States in her day.

The Chi Masters of China.

They are too numerous to list here. I had the wonderful experience of studying under them during my too short stay in China. It would take many life times to learn all they had to offer. They opened many doors for me, giving me a different view of how the mind and body work together.

Betty Currie, M.S.ED

She never considered herself a healer because she was so infirm of body, yet she used her experience to teach others great things. The first five years of her life were normal. She was a happy child filled with unbelievable curiosity. One morning she woke up and could not move. She spent the next 5 years in an "Iron Lung" at a Shiners Hospital in Canada. Then she lived at home in her wheelchair until she was an adult. Not being able to move it by her self, she depended on the neighborhood kids to push her through the woods and fields and across the streams getting into as much or more trouble then the rest. She was always the instigator! It was many years before they found out she had a very rare form of childhood rheumatoid arthritis. In later years she could use crutches in a "walking doll way", not being able to use her knees & hips. I met her during her stay in a convalescent center when I was in my 30's. I was her nurse. She could not reach her head, her feet or her seat. She was totally dependent on others for her life. But she went anywhere anyone would take her including riding a motorcycle. Even with her disability she had an active romantic life with much joy.

She finished collage with a degree in English and Future Studies. Going to collage was the first time she had ever been in a school. She taught herself to read backwards through the mirror from her Iron Lung, as a child. She traveled the world and wrote several books and produced training sessions on patient care, all without being able to bend her elbows or flex her fingers. She spent all of her life in a wheelchair, or flat on her back after she was in her 20's. She embraced the idea of keeping a sense of humor writing articles like, "Arthur Itis, My Constant Companion", "Belt Buckle & Fly", The View of The World From a Wheel Chair. Or "Up Your Nose. My View From a Hospital Bed."

These people did not start out to become healers. Their compassion for humanity lead them there. Being a healer may not mean saving a life in the traditional sense. It can mean offering a smile, a pat, touch, hug, a kind word to any one you see. It is a positive exchange of energy between you, Your Higher Power and the person you are relating to. It is making a change. You will never know how much your small token may change a life, including yours. But unless you are as healthy as you can be, you won't have the energy or positive motivation to pass it on. Above all, we are here for each other.

May Asclepius be with you all.

Contents

Foreword ix
Healers I have known.. xiii
Chapter 1 Who, What, Why & Water..................1
Chapter 2 Measured Breathing.......................... 11
Chapter 3 Meditation 17
Chapter 4 Reflexology for Hands and Feet.......25
Chapter 5 Our Thymus Gland...........................31
Chapter 6 Tapping for Health. 37
Chapter 7 5 Treasures QiGong,
               Simple steps everyone can do. 47
Chapter 8 Sleep, Why We Need It! 59
Chapter 9 Sounds of Life 67
Biography 69
Bibliography 73

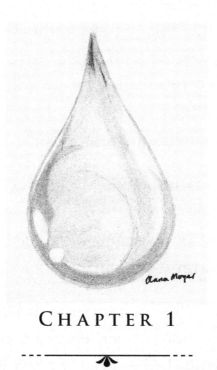

CHAPTER 1

Who, What, Why & Water

The information in this book is empowering and will change your life forever. You can follow the directions just as they are written. You don't need to take an expensive class, buy a product, or change your belief system.

We offer this life saving information in easy to follow steps. Nothing more to buy, ever. Share with your family of any age and condition. Children love to be involved with you as you practice these 7 easy steps. Elders are able to incorporate these steps into their everyday living with little effort. No more gym fees to pay. No tapes, gadgets or questionable pills to buy- ever. Many have taken these 7 simple steps into their lives with amazing results.

As more and more people are taking on increasing responsibility for the state of their own health and that of loved ones, learning holistic health modalities is becoming a must do, now and for the future.

The days of 100% employer-provided health insurance are gone forever. We don't know what the future will bring. Today, according to AARP's latest figures, there are approximately 46.7 million people with no health insurance and many who have no access to affordable medical care. Even those with good insurance polices are finding to their horror that many procedures they believed were covered are not.

Isn't it better to take control of your own health care as much as possible? Seeing your health care provider as a partner working together with you to keep you well?

We're not trying to take the place of your medical care provider nor in any way suggest that you don't need one. Our goal is to educate you about activities you can do, for free, to help you and your family have and maintain a healthy pain -free life. You will have less trips to your doctor with a little fun at the same time!

Of course it goes without saying, that you should do everything you can to stay in as healthy an environment as you possibly can. You can learn which foods are best for you and your family. You can discover how much restful sleep you really need and make decisions on how you can make that happen.

You can decide what activities are the most beneficial for you and your family and learn how to live in balanced relationships. Even on the most stringent budget, most of us can make better choices, if we believe we can.

There is free information about nutrition, exercise, relationships and how our body functions available in libraries and on web sites free of charge. We live in a time in which free life-changing information is available to virtually everyone, if they want it. There is no reason why you shouldn't educate yourself to create the healthiest and most enjoyable environment possible, inside and out. We are not talking about the latest fad, but helping you learn what is truly healthy for you and your family on every level. Many of us work several jobs or have the stress of being out of work. People and animals we love die, leaving us in emotional turmoil. These situations are real and can be very frustrating and scary. The steps we describe here are not meant to sugar coat real life situations or make them seem light and fluffy. You can not control what anyone else says, does or believes. You can only control your own choices if you realize you have them, and then you can control **YOUR** behavior.

We live in that snug package we call our body with a mind capable of shining light, both inside and out, as well as traveling the universe of unimaginable creative ideas, steered by our emotions with Spirit connecting the two. We are truly remarkable and we are meant to be healthy and happy.

I know you have all heard the phrase, "Listen to your body" Like you can find time to do **THAT**, what ever that means. Every cell of your body is a whole living being on its own. Each cell of your body whether they form your eyelids, liver, or hair, can and do communicate with each other, and with you as a whole. Our life today is non stop, from the time we wake up until we sleep. The sound of our living is too great to hear without a lot of mindful effort. We need to make time for quiet every day, even if only for 15 minutes at a time.

As in anything, use common sense. See a doctor when common sense says you need to. You will not set a broken leg with Tapping or Emotional Freedom Technique, (EFT) cure cancer with meditation alone, reduce psoriasis with massage or heal pneumonia with structured breathing! But you can learn how to stay healthier with the practices that follow. They will have a positive effect on your mental, physical, emotional and spiritual health. If you are currently on medication or in any type of therapy, please do not stop what you are doing without first consulting your doctor. Part of listening to your body includes noticing how we are breathing. Is your breath smooth and clear or short and choppy? Do you have a headache or a niggling pain in your neck? Ask your self why. How are your bowels ? Do you go regular according to your food intake? If not, how often do you have problems? Take note of color, smell and consistency that may be different from time to time. These are all noticeable ways your body tells you that there may be a health issue. There are many illnesses that are silent. They may sneak up on you, even if you are doing your best to stay connected. Ovarian and Kidney cancer are two of the more sneaky ones. There is no pain or other symptoms until very late in the process. So the more you pay attention to all of your life style, and general health the better off you will be.

This book is about living as well and as mindfully as you can by paying attention to your choices, your body and your happiness. It is also about developing a good medical team who can get to know you and what you believe in.

We will introduce you to 7 basic modalities that are simple to learn, life enhancing and free. These modalities start at the most basic. Just about everyone will be able to understand and follow through with the ideas that interest them most. As you learn and enjoy, you might want to enhance your own learning for yourself, or become fully trained in a modality that you can share with others. Here you might want to start a new practice each week or each month, depending on what schedule works for you. Work with the same practice each day until you are comfortable with one, then add another. Do two practice sessions each day until you are comfortable with those and so on ...

Slowly add one at a time until you can do all seven each day or several days each week. Bringing friends or children into your actives will add fun and laughter, which in turn releases stress, clears your mind and sets a positive tone for the rest of the day. One of the most important things you can do for your health at any time is to keep hydrated. Your body and all of it's working parts work with fluid and the nutrients in water as well as the electric flow between them.

Water is the conductor of our electrical current. This came racing home to me one day last year. I have rarely ever been sick. Haven't had a flu or cold in many years. It was the mid-summer heat of July in Oklahoma. I had been in the garden most of the afternoon. I had started feeling sick to my stomach. I went inside thinking I may have picked up some stomach bug. I didn't feel much better the next day. I for sure had something. Who goes to the doctor for a stomach flu? So, I just buckled down and figured I would just deal with going both ends. I drank more water and other liquids. Well, a couple of weeks later I was still feeling ill. My husband had a fit, and I insisted I see my doctor. Well, who goes to the doctor for a stomach flu? Long story short, I went. After appropriate blood work, he came back into the room with a strange look on his face. I asked jokingly if I was going to die. He went white as a ghost, said that my kidneys were shutting down, and that I had about 24 hours to live!

Had I not gone in I may have just been found dead in my bed, with no one knowing why. I had gotten way over dehydrated without realizing it. I knew better but... I had been drinking more, but not enough. I did figure that something was wrong when my urine output had nearly stopped. But by that time I couldn't think straight and didn't know it.

Dehydration is a serious issue for everyone but especially older people and small children. By the time a child asks for a drink they may have already started to dehydrate. Elders may not know or remember that they didn't have enough to drink. They may not know that they don't drink enough and those who care for them may not realize it either. Often forgetfulness is due to lack of hydration. Re-hydration is not just about drinking water. Jell-O, ice cream, soup and popsicles are liquid and can help to add fluid to your system.

I was put on intravenous fluids immediately. I was better in a few weeks. All systems were go. It took me nearly six months to recover my strength and vitality. Oh, I was up and around and doing everything, but it took me some time to get my oomph back. I really did not know how sick I was. I had no idea that I was dying. How do you know you may be dead in 24 hours from a medical issue you have no idea you had? I did have a "near death experience" when I was a child, but it was nothing like this. I don't know if anyone would call this a near death experience. But I guess if it was, I was near. Now I make sure I drink all the time... water that is. Alcohol and caffeine will dehydrate you more. Check the labels of what you chose to drink, specially sports drinks. Often they have much more sugar and caffeine than is healthy. They may cause you problems if you are diabetic as well. I just carry a water bottle with me everywhere I go. Simple. Works for me!

The first thing I would like to introduce you to is breathing. Ok, I know you do it, but...

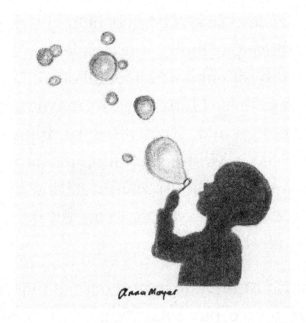

CHAPTER 2

---✥---

Measured Breathing

Measured or structured breathing is simple to learn. The way you breathe can reduce your pain, increase your sense of relaxation, lower your blood pressure, increase the blood flow and oxygen to your lungs and heart, as well as increase your physical and emotional energy. Our body is made up of trillions and trillions of microscopic cells. When they can not get enough oxygen they become depleted, causing you to feel tired and exhausted. Eventually causing you to become sick. Oxygen helps us digest our food, to move our limbs, muscles, keeping us alive. To be healthy, it's important for all of our body parts to work together. Think back to maybe when you were a young child. Remember running through the fields like a wild horse, jumping into the lake and swimming like a fish, never getting tired? You were there once. Maybe you can get back to that wonderful feeling.

Most of us just breathe in and out without thought. We only notice our breathing rhythm when it's difficult for us to take in air, like when we are ill, have allergies, or when our system is stressed and we are scared or very upset. Then we tend to hold our breath. As soon as we relax, we feel the relief in our shoulders as our normal rhythm starts again. Using your breath to consciously calm yourself or to control pain is as simple as learning the steps and remembering them.

Hold your breath as long as you can, then let go. Notice how your body feels when you hold your breath, and when you inhale again.

Breathing is something you were born to do. You have been breathing since the moment you were born. Your breath is your life essence. You will breath in and out approximately 714,861,000 times. (That's seven hundred fourteen million, eight hundred and sixty-one thousand!) Almost a billion times during your life span. If Bill Gates gave you $2.00 for every breath you took during your life time, he would still have over half his fortune left!

Your ability to breathe controls the amount of oxygen needed to operate your bodily functions. If you cut the amount of oxygen going to your lungs by being in a polluted air environment, by smoking, or through an illness, you directly effect the oxygen going into your bloodstream, lungs, heart, muscles and brain, lowering the ability to function in all your organs. Without proper air, you lose your ability to think clearly, handle emotional stress, digest your food or even move your limbs. If you stop breathing, you will die in approximately 4 minutes.

Your first step is simple. Shut off your phone and try to have no interruptions for 15 minutes. Slowly breath in through your nose to the silent count of 4. Then slowly breath out through your mouth to the to the silent count of 4. Practice for 15 minuets in the morning and 15 minuets in the afternoon or evening. Increase your practice until you are comfortable doing this several times a day, each day. (I set a kitchen timer so I know I have somewhere near the correct time.) Then see if you can train yourself to do conscious breathing once or twice when something or someone ticks you off. See how easy it is to calm down? This will help you keep your blood pressure even and calm and your mind clear. Doing this will give you time before your jump into a fray, or say something you will regret. As this breathing becomes second nature to you several times a day, this practice will reduce your anxiety, fear, pain and anger, among many other benefits. Did you know that only a relaxed breath can blow bubbles? When your breath is ragged or harsh you will pop the delicate tension that holds the bubble together.

Be happy when you sing. Make a joyful noise, be happy! Singing opens the chest and lengthens and compresses your diaphragm, forcing oxygen through your system. Singing connects you with your emotional well-being as well. Have you ever been able to stay angry when you were singing? Laughing does the same and maybe does it better. It is said laughter is the best medicine. Laughing is like giving yourself an internal massage! All of your innards kind of bounce around and hug each other. When was the last time you had a good belly laugh? What made you laugh? You can't stay in a bad mood when you're laughing. Try it! Laughter is natures best medicine. Laughing increases your oxygen intake. Laughter creates endorphins that help you reduce pain, reduce depression and makes people around you feel more at ease. Besides, if you are laughing, people will wonder what you're up to! Keep a small jar of bubbles in your car or purse. When you are stuck in traffic, just blow 'em out the window! We did that once crossing a bridge in N.Y. City. The traffic was stopped. The next thing we knew a big burly truck driver crawled by, waving to us and singing "Tiny Bubbles"!! It changed the attitude of the whole bridge!

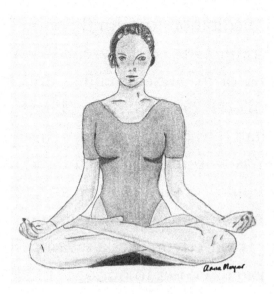

Chapter 3

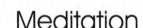

Meditation

In 1972 Wallace and Benson, in their study of the physiology of meditation, noted that a specific set of physiological changes (an integrated response) occurred during meditation. It represented a quiescence of the sympathetic nervous system. In other words, it seemed to be an integrated response that was essentially opposite to the integrated "fight or flight" response in that regular meditation has an effect on your fight or fight response. Many of the greatest thinkers and geniuses in our history have used meditation to calm the mind and vision with the brain. One of the greatest was DaVinci. He was one of greatest inventors and artists and medical explorers on earth so far. There was Nikola Tesla. He had the ability to envision his diagrams in meditation as working in his head and understand how they could be put together and work in real time. All of the non wireless communication we use today is based on Tesla's work. There was Albert Einstein. Closer to our own time. He called his meditation "brain wanderings". He "saw" and "learned" the math language of the universe through his meditation. We may not all have the ability to be an Einstein, but we all have the ability to calm our minds and use them to help and heal us at every level.

Meditation is a way to quiet the mind and soul. The mental calmness that regular meditation provides can give you space to think and to connect with your Creator. It offers the opportunity to listen for the answers we often ask for. Meditation is easy to learn and because the ability to meditate is connected to your breath, you carry the possibilities of peacefulness within you, 24/7.

Meditation is not about blotting out the world. It's about becoming a vehicle for bringing the highest good to ourselves, mind, body and Spirit and to the world we live in.

We set aside time for the replenishment of our body, we sleep and eat so that our body can heal and rejuvenate itself from the day's work. Most of us do not set aside regular quiet time for our soul (meditation). Some of the benefits of meditation are self-healing at all levels, clear vision for dealing with problem solving and decision making, lowered blood pressure, and as a focus point to send healing to others, also called prayer. In the practice of meditation, or deep prayer, the phantoms of the mind are swept away. I try to set aside 15 minutes a day for just being quiet. No TV, no phone, no nothing. I set my kitchen timer, put it under a pillow in the next room so that the bell doesn't jump me out of my skin when it goes off. I can hear it quietly go off. Some days I make it and some days I don't. Some days I take my 15 minutes to just be still or work on a problem looking for insight and other times I take this time to be in prayer. There is some effort in learning to be quiet and alone, even for 15 minutes. Our world is not set up in this day and age for us to learn how. But once learned and comfortable with the practice, I promise you will want to make this part of your every day life.

I am like everyone else. Some days I follow many of these practices and other days not so much.

Each of us has a different lifestyle, time schedule, and metabolism. What works in one person's life may not work for another. It stands to reason that people might find different methods of meditation that are appropriate for them. Aids such as candles, incense, music, stones, spiritual affirmations and chanting, are used by some. These tools may help to still and focus your mind, or perhaps to trigger a memory pattern which could well help in unraveling a persistent problem. But aids are only aids. They are not the source of the stillness we are looking for.

There are many ways to meditate. Develop what works best for you. Some people are more comfortable concentrating on a single point, like a flower or a flame or a mantra (a repetition of words or sounds used to still the mind.). Others visualize their own or another's body and mind being healthy and full of light, read helpful passages from the Bible or other sacred text. Many people learn to focus on the rhythm of their breath. Breathing is fundamental! By learning to focus on your breath, you can learn to still your mind as well.

At the end of your meditation time you might want to give thanks for the blessings that you have. Sometimes we forget what they are. Giving thanks helps us stay mindful as we go about our busy lives. As we become more mindful day to day we find that we feel better as our pain level and blood pressure are often lowered.

Meditation can bring a different view of the world, one with compassion. You begin to see a world that is truly about love and that we are all interconnected. This world view fosters hope and mutual understanding and well-being to our body, mind and spirit.

Although the approach to meditation, and the results, may differ, the same understanding, the same point of consciousness and the same state of awareness are still the ultimate goals of individuals who use this practice. We believe prayer is the act of asking our Creator for the things we need or want as well as giving thanks; meditation is listening for the answers, seeking the answers through the stilling of our minds.

To enter a state of meditation, let your body become utterly relaxed, allowing your tension to flow from your body as well as your mind. Use whatever methods work for you - conscious breathing, listening to music, star gazing, slowly walking through your garden or through the woods. Being mindful of what there is around you no matter how tiny, doing any activity that helps you feel safe and comfortable.

Take a minute to close your eyes and envision yourself alone in a house that you don't know well, like baby-sitting or care-taking the property or something similar. There is a raging storm outside. As the lights flicker your stomach starts to knot, you start getting nervous, your palms may start to sweat your, breathing and heart becomes more rapid. The lights and TV go out with a horrific clap of thunder and lightning that emanates throughout the house for seconds that feel like minutes. The storm rages on. You hear something. You are not sure what. Branches are banging against the house along with some other unidentified sound. You think someone might be breaking in. You have about had it. You are scared. Your heart is racing, your entire body breaks out in a cold sweat, you are shaking. You find the flashlight and grab the kitchen broom, pulling up every bit of courage you have, trying not to throw up, you creep into the next room ready to clobber any one who is there.

To your shock and total relief, it's only the cat playing with its toy. With a loud HA!, You let out the breath you were holding. You even start to laugh at your own silliness. Your heart and breath slow back to normal, your stomach has calmed. With the flashlight you round up some candles and are set for the evening.

Millennia ago, back in cave times, our fight or flight response kept us alive. With all systems on go, we had to decide quickly if we were going to fight the thing that was after us or run as fast as our legs would carry us.

In the world we live in today our fight or flight response is triggered many times a day. We are programmed on "screech" most of the time. The constant revving of our motor wears our systems out. We become sick, depressed and crabby. We are overtired from running on high speed constantly. Meditation is a way to quiet our systems down.

Once you learn how, you can call on this quietness any time you need it to bring clarity in order to make good decisions and chose which behavior is appropriate for the situation.

Allow yourself quiet time of about 5 minutes to start. Do the breathing you have learned and place your focus on your steady breathing in and out. Once you are comfortable with 5 minutes, add an evening or afternoon quiet session. Ad more time as you are comfortable each day until you can get to 20 minutes once a day, then twice a day. Stay with the breathing and meditation for as long as you are comfortable, until you are ready for your next step. As you will see, even if you stay with only the breathing for some time, it will make a great difference in your health at all levels. It may be a good time to teach your loved ones that this can be quiet time for every one.

The Path of the Compassionate Spirit is one many of us strive for in our spiritual development as we work to be in harmony with and connected to the Universe.

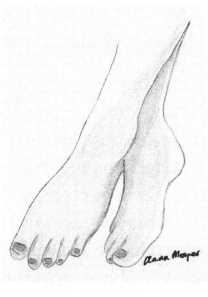

CHAPTER 4

---✼---

Reflexology for Hands and Feet

Did you know that your skin is the largest organ of your body? Your skin covers every part of you and was functioning even before you were born. Your skin helps your body release toxins, keeps you cool, feels pleasure or pain, and sends all of this information to your brain. It helps you define your world in many ways. Its color can help diagnose health or illness. Your skin holds you in a cocoon keeping you alive. You would surely be a funny looking critter if you went around without skin!

We have thousands of places on our skin that have what we call "pressure points". Many cultures believe that these pressure points are related to inner organs throughout your body. The Chinese call these points acupuncture points. Chinese acupuncture is thousands of years old and done with hair thin needles that are not painful. There are many physicians and chiropractors in this country who use this method as part of their wellness system. Acupuncture without needles is called acupressure or reflexology. Points on the hands, feet or ears are the easiest to use. Reflexology or foot massage have some of the easiest points to learn and remember. You can do this to relieve simple pain or stress on yourself or family. Acupressure is very helpful and is not painful to do. Although some rflexologists believe that a very firm pressure is better, we believe that a medium pressure that is not painful and done several times over is more beneficial. More firm pressure can be added along the way by using the thumb or an implement like a the end of a pencil eraser. While helpful, this harder pressure also puts stress on the body as your skin and muscles respond to pain, your body tenses and causes more pain to be felt. In our opinion, light pressure moving toward a firmer pressure is better than painful stabbing! As you become more and more comfortable performing these moves on yourself or family, your body will relax so that you will be more comfortable using more pressure.

On the next few pages you will find a simple outline of a hand and a foot with reflex points. Use these pages to guide you. There are excellent books on reflexology on line or in your local library that will give you a larger overview.

You can start slowly with gently squeezing the points on each finger, than the palm of you hand. One then the other. Do both hands. Try different levels of pressure, from soft to medium and harder, but not hurting. Do each hand every day until it's comfortable for you. Then start on your feet. If your feet are hard to reach use a foot roller or a thick soda bottle. Again, do it each day until you feel comfortable doing it. As you work, you will find that there may be a difference in your pain or discomfort levels for the better. Remember that this outline is very basic instruction. When you do reflexology you are not just pushing skin around.

You are feeling under the skin for little bumps or something feeling like bits of sand. Then you will rub in a circular motion over these points until they disappear. Sometimes it takes several tries to get the hang of it. You will. Don't worry. You will earn as you go along.

If you find this useful, you can get more information to teach yourself, or find a Reflexologist in your area. There are also hundreds of acupressure spots in your ears and all over your body.

Reflexology is a way you can help someone who you may not be able to touch in any other way. If someone is in the hospital or very ill, gently rubbing their hands or feet will give them a great sense of peace and caring. It will help them to feel loved and wanted. The way we touch brings us into our humanness with no barriers. We can give, and we can find a way to pass on the caring without words. Even if you think a loved one may not hear you or feel what you are doing for them, they do. The soul always knows. In the end, all we want or need is love. This is a simple way to show it.

The charts are for you to review. You can practice hand and foot reflexology and massage just by feel. I have taught blind students in my massage classes. In China, only the blind were allowed to do massage. I don't know if that has changed or not. It was a lot of years ago.

You can find these easy yo use charts on the internet. Many of them are free.

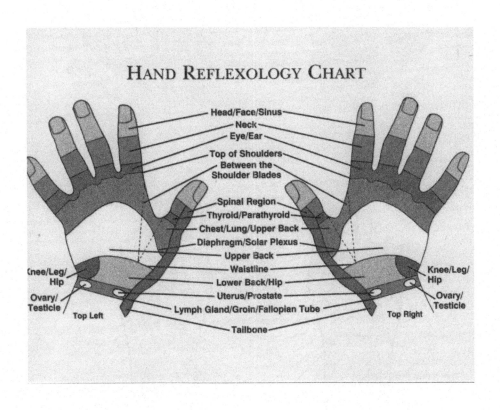

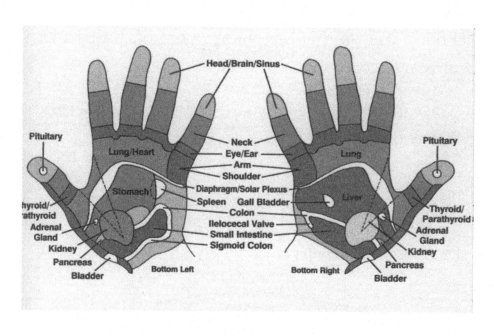
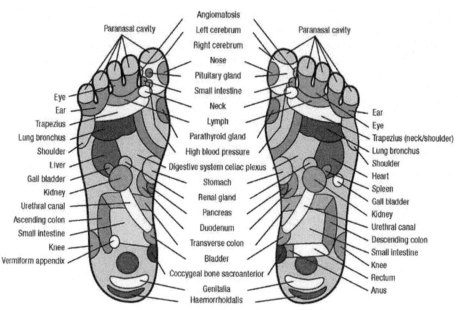

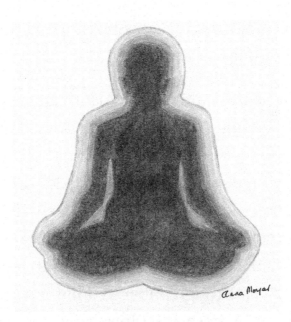

CHAPTER 5

Our Thymus Gland

Even though these exercises don't have anything directly to do with our thymus, you will find it will have everything to do with it in some way. We could not live without it or hormones replacing it. Ever hear of the admonition, "think happy thoughts"? Find peace in beauty or positive pleasing music? I guess you could call our thymus our "happy gland". It is very responsible for our well being and over all health. It is vitally important to keep to keep our thymus as stress free as possible so that it will continue to help us stay well.

Our thymus is located just beneath the upper part of our breast bone in the middle of our chest. Over 100 years ago physicians were using thymus extract in the treatment of cancer. It was widely believed by physicians of the time that after puberty the thymus had no function, because in autopsies of infants of the time their thymus was larger than that of a child who had gone through puberty. Thus it was thought to be a gland whose usefulness was only found in infants, helping them grow.

By the 1950's pathologists took note of the fact that battlefield autopsies during the Korean War revealed that soldiers who died in battle had larger thymus glands then men of the same age who died from "natural causes". Eventually it was realized that the thymus shrinks rapidly during serious illness or great physical stress.

In a person whose thymus gland has been removed or destroyed, there is a loss in effectiveness of the immune systems of the body that guard against infection and cancerous growth. However, if the thymus gland is intact and healthy, then the tumor will be recognized as a hostile invader and will be rejected. Before birth and in early life the thymus gland is concerned with growth. But more importantly, it is the school and factory for lymphocytes - the white blood cells responsible for the immunological reactions in the body. Lymphocytes, in an immature state, come to the thymus from our bone marrow. Under the influence of thymus hormones, these cells mature, then leave the thymus and settle in the lymph nodes and the spleen, where they produce other generations of lymphocytes called T cells.

When your mom or your doctor checked the glands under the sides of your jaw or your underarms when you were small they were checking to see if your glands were swollen, to see if you might have an infection that the lymphocytes (white blood cells) were trying to fight off. The thymus can be considered to be a true endocrine gland - that is an organ that secretes a hormone into the bloodstream to be carried to another part of the body where it will have its effect. The thymus continues to train and export T cells until very late in life. After puberty your thymus gets smaller because it no longer needs to help your body grow. It is now concerned with keeping you healthy.

To know the difference between self from not self, friend from foe, and to destroy foreign cells. Any further shrinkage is due to stress, physical, mental, emotional or spiritual.

Today it is known that of all the billions and billions of new cells produced each day, some will be abnormal. One of the functions of the T cells is to find and destroy the abnormal ones. But if the T cells are not activated by the thymus hormone, the abnormal cells may 'take' and develop into a type of cancer. I am in no way suggesting that Thymus hormone therapy will cure you of cancer. Only that taking care of your health will help you in many areas of your life, throughout your lifetime.

All of the exercises in this book help in part to keep your thymus strong and healthy. One more thing you can do, even though it may sound and look silly is, when you are feeling upset, vulnerable, tired, scared, or stressed, take in a deep slow breath and let it out while you gently tap over the area of your thymus gland. Three or four thumps is all that is needed. Do it whenever you think about it. Upset with someone? Tap. Stressed out because of bills, breathe and tap. It won't pay your bills, but will clear your mind, help you relax and perhaps think of other ways to solve the problem. One of the phrases I often use when tapping or quiet meditation is, "Be still and know that I am God".

Chapter 6

Tapping for Health.

Tapping for Health is also called Emotional Freedom Technique. It is a combination of visualization, tapping and affirmations, developed by Gary Craig. There is also books written by Nick Ortner, The Tapping Solution for Pain Relief. You can find this information in the back of this book.

You can learn to tap on any issue when you are in pain, fear, or discomfort of any kind. Tapping can help you lose weight, stop smoking, remove the fear of spiders and flying, as well as improve your golf game. Really! It does work! EFT has been used to work through the issues associated with PTSD. This outline has been added because it is easy to learn and is very helpful in many areas. We want to remind you that if you feel you are having a serious problem with any physical or emotional issues, contact your doctor or other health care provider. Even though we have worked with many hundreds of people who recognize the value and helpfulness that tapping can have, do not try to self diagnose. If you break your leg you would go to a doctor to have X Rays and have it set if needed. You might be given pain medication. EFT will help you reduce the pain so you may not need to take as much pain medication. It also may help you recover from the emotional trauma of breaking a bone and the situation surrounding the incident but, tapping alone will not set or heal your leg. In other words, use common sense.

The theory of Tapping or Emotional Freedom Technique (EFT) is based on the Eastern medical idea that within your body, lines of energy run through what are called meridians. Meridians can't be seen; they are part of the connection of matter and Spirit which work together forming the whole. EFT works through a series of memorized affirmations and rapid tapping procedures applied to the ends of the basic meridians, mostly on face and hands, closing the gap of the energy disruption. The tapping procedure is the centerpiece of EFT. It is the primary tool for "emotional freedom". It may look funny and feel silly, but the results are profound.

EFT works the same as acupuncture and acupressure, painlessly tapping into our energy system and removing barriers or blockages caused by emotional trauma. This results in emotional freedom or clarity, assisting the physical body to heal as the emotional/spiritual trauma is healed. EFT is known to reduce or eliminate many causes of pain.

How to practice Tapping for Health on yourself

People are using "Tapping" to stop smoking, lose weight, subdue pain, work through grief, and to quell anxiety and fear in many areas of their lives. Many people are using these techniques to recover from a variety of Post Traumatic Stress Disorder (PTSD) issues as well. Tapping works through a series of memorized affirmations and rapid tapping procedures applied to the ends of basic meridians, primarily on the face and face and hands, closing the gap of energy disruption. This tapping process is the center piece of EFT. It is the primary tool "Emotional Freedom Technique'. At first it may look funny or feel silly, but the positive results are profound.

DISCLAIMER: *Tapping is gentle and easy to use, and has yielded remarkable results for relieving emotional and physical distress. While there have been no distressing side-effects reported, this does not mean you will not discover side-effects yourself. If you use this method of self help, you agree to hold Healing Focus, Gary Craig, Author House or any of our associates free from harm.*

Tapping also called Emotional Freedom Technique (EFT) developed by Gary Craig, is about tapping into the affirmation of your own truth. The closer you can get to that kernel, the better EFT works. This information is found free on line at www.emofree.com

EFT is a process of "tuning in" while balancing the body's energy system.

EFT works best on specific events or pain.

EFT will hold true even when done "out of context", such as fear of flying while sitting in your living room.

EFT works progressively. (Taking down one tree at a time, eventually the whole forest is gone).

Addictive substances are a means of "tranquilizing anxiety"(chocolate, cigarettes, drugs, food, alcohol). EFT will work on these issues once you have located the core of your issue.

Recently, I fell out of a tree and injured my knee. It's a long story. Don't ask. (I was born in 1946) After X-rays, it was suggested that I had a torn meniscus. I used EFT to help reduce the pain. It worked well. I was in a knee brace for four weeks and on pain medication for two. EFT did not heal my knee, but it did reduce the pain and helped me feel less frantic. I didn't need surgery or any other medical care except to follow my doctors suggestions and advice. When something happens in my life to stress me out a great deal, I practice all of the suggestions in this book one at a time. They work in different ways, with different people and also people of different ages. A six year old child will have a different response than a 40 year old man. All these ideas together work in different ways. Please don't assume that any one practice will cure what ails you. But together they may make a much more pleasant life for you and your

The Process

Read each sentence slowly, one at a time. Once you get the hang of it you will be able to move through more quickly. Don't worry about it.

Step 1. Rate your discomfort on a scale from 1-10.

Step 2. The setup: Repeat this affirmation 3 times while continuously tapping the Karate Chop point. (Fleshy side of hand, where pinky attaches to hand.)

Step 3. Tapping face sequence

Step 4. The 9 Gamut movements

Step 5. Eye movements, humming & counting. The original process I learned from Gary included humming and eye movements. I have found that the process works just as well if I don't include them

Step 6. Check scale from 0-10. If discomfort remains, do shortened version of the face tapping sequence.

Step 7. Repeat process until scale of discomfort is at 0.

The Basic recipe

Step 1. Rate your discomfort on a scale from 0-10.

Step 2. The setup: Repeat this affirmation 3 times while continuously tapping the Karate Chop point. (Fleshy side of hand where pinky attaches to hand).

"Even though I have this *feeling of anxiety*" (or whatever you are feeling), "I deeply and completely accept myself".

The Sequence: Tap about 7 times on the end of each of the following energy points while repeating the **Reminder Phrase**, "even though I have or feel this..."

Tapping points : **EB** - eyebrow, **SE** - side of eye, **UE** - under eye, **UN** - under nose, **CH** - chin, **MC**- upper chest (thymus area), **UA**- under arm, **TH** - top of head.

Step 3. Check your scale from 0 - 10. If you are not at 0, do the 9 Gamut procedure below with the eye movements, humming and counting. If you are still in discomfort, start the face tapping again with the abbreviated version of your setup. (Remaining pain, etc.) Go through the process as often as you need to get to a more comfortable level, or follow the same process that you have just done and substitute the words, I choose......

"I choose to to be free of this pain in my shoulder..."

Step 4. The 9 Gamut

Tap side of TH - thumb, side of **IF** -Index finger, side of **MF** - middle finger, side of **PF** - pinky finger, then back of hand between ring and index finger, while doing eye movements, humming, then counting to five rapidly.

Step 5. Check your comfort scale of 0 -10. If you are still in discomfort, start the face tapping again, with the abbreviated version of your setup. (remaining pain). Go through the process as often as necessary to reach comfortable levels.

Yes, I know this sounds crazy, but it really works for most issues with most people. We have had tremendous results for people with PTSD and many different pain issues, fear of flying, fear of water and bugs, weight loss and smoking addictions. Try it on everything. It won't hurt you and may make you and those around you laugh out loud!

Chapter 7

5 Treasures QiGong, Simple steps everyone can do.

Some forms of meditation also include things like Qi Gong, a moving type of meditation. Anyone can do a slow physical movements paired with slow breathing. These exercises will bring oxygen to your system, clarity to your mind and a gentle flexibility to your body by gradually warming the synovial fluid in your joints. As you get used to following these steps you will find your body to be more flexible and less painful. If you are disabled in any way you can still do many of these movements with the parts of your body that work the best for you. Qi Gong will help reduce your blood pressure, lowering anger and frustration. It will give you a pleasant outlook on life no matter what your circumstances are. The kids, even as young as 2-3 years love to exercise with you. Put on some slow music and watch them try to copy what you do. That will get you laughing like nothing else. I was taught Qi Gong when I studied in China. Groups of men and women would form a circle every morning in the park, about 6 am. I was honored one morning as I was watching, by one of the woman coming to take my hand and lead me to the circle. I didn't speak Chines and she didn't speak English. She showed me step by step how to go slowly through the gentle movements without music. I felt like I was dancing an intricate ballet in a flowing sea of birds. Feel free to add music. I do. It helps me keep on a smooth pace, opens my breathing and calms me. Even though I have been teaching Qigong for over 20 years I have not made a DVD. You can purchase one with a donation from the National Qigong Association. NQA is a non-profit organization. They offer beautiful easy to follow DVD's of the "5 Treasures" Their contact information is listed in the back of this book. I am not associated with NQA in any way except to purchase their DVD's for my classes.

Discovering the 5 Treasures Qigong

A simple outline developed by the National Qigong Association. Qigong is the skill of cultivating vital energy. Qigong integrates physical postures and breathing techniques with focused intention. There are three major schools of Qigong: Medical, Martial and Spiritual. It's great appeal is that everyone can benefit, regardless of ability, age, and belief systems or life circumstances.

FIVE TREASURES PRACTICE SET

This practice set is designed to work with the overall energy of the body. Keep in mind when practicing the moves that they can be modified to fit your individual circumstances. The set should be performed within a comfortable range for you. This practice set is divided into three sections: 1. Warm-up (for cleansing) 2. Five treasures Set (Collecting and circulating energy) and 3. Closing (storing energy)

Warmups (Cleansing)

* SHAKE THE TREE

Begin by relaxing the entire body as you shake loose any tension or tightness. Feel your joints open allowing for the energy channels to open, feeling a release of any blocked energy in your entire body, including your internal organs. Shake and vibrate the body in unison.

* TWIST FROM THE WAIST, SWING YOUR ARMS

This move begins by shifting the body weight left and right while simultaneously twisting the waist. Allow for for the arms to swing naturally, tapping gently in the front and back of the waist.

Keep the hands in a soft fist. This stimulates the kidney meridians as well as the belt channel in particular, and the energy on the left and right sides of the body.

*CENTERING POSITION

This position is done from a relaxed, natural standing posture. Stand with your spine erect and relaxed, feet and knees facing forward with arms down and the palms facing below the navel. This is a neutral position for centering and grounding and is used to transition between movements as well as beginning and ending a sequence.

FIVE TREASURES SET (collecting and circulating the energy)

* OCEAN WAVE BREATHING

Begin from the centering position. Using the image of standing in the ocean, imagine waves coming up gently pushing your hands upward as your entire body rocks gently forward and backward. As you inhale, allow your hands to rise up in front of your body slightly. As you exhale, bring your hands back as your entire body relaxes and sinks. As you continue to inhale and exhale, make your arm motions larger & larger. Breathe slowly and evenly in coordination with your movements. Gradually slow down and return to smaller movements. End in the centering position.

* DRAW UP EARTH QI

From the centering position, use the image of scooping up the Earth energy, raise up the body stretching the arms and palms towards the heavens, as you inhale. as you exhale, squat slightly, turning your palms down towards the Earth. Focus on the whole body movement, feeling the energy of reaching up and sinking down. Repeat several times, ending in the centering position.

* GATHERING IN STARLIGHT

From the centering position, use the image of your energy body expanding in the vastness of the universe and connect with the stars. At the same time step out with the right foot while reaching up with your right hand, place your left hand in the middle of your lower back, (opposite of your navel) holding five fingertips together at the same point. Begin to circle the right hand towards the heavens, collecting starlight, as you shift your weight forward and backward. Repeat several times as you bring this energy down from your head, then your heart, then your abdomen.

Focus on gathering the energy and circulating it through your body, to nourish your soul. Switch to the left side and repeat. Return to your centering position.

* OPEN YOUR HEART

Begin in the centering position. Using the image o gathering energy into your heart, as you inhale reach forward with your arms puling the energy directly into your heart center of your chest. Relax your body as you repeat this several times. Then reverse the direction as you exhale, while you reach forward extending the hands palms facing upward from your heart as a symbol of giving and sharing. Feel all your emotional and mental obstacles and let go. Repeat several times.

* DRAW DOWN HEAVEN QI

From the centering position, use the image of drawing heaven energy down through your body. as you inhale, reach toward the heavens connecting with the energy above. As you exhale, lower your hands, bringing the heaven qi down through the top of your head into your chest, abdomen, legs and out through your feet. Feel the energy collecting circulating, circulating and illuminating your entire body. Repeat several times.

CLOSING (Storing energy)

STORING AND SMOOTHING THE QI

Begin by using your palm to brush down the inside of your right arm, from your shoulder down and off the finger tips. Repeat this with the left arm. Then brush down the inside and outside and then the front and back, of each leg from the hips down to the toes. Then use your palms to brush energy down the front of your chest, from your throat to your abdomen. Finally, placing your palms over each other circle your palms/ hands over your abdomen in a clockwise position. Feel the energy naturally permeate through your entire body. You may hold this position for a few minutes to complete the practice session.

By starting a daily routine, it is said that you may be able to regain your vitally, good health and promote longevity and recover from illness. Qi Gong harmonizes the body, mind an soul connections.

As we have said in other places in this book. This information is meant to be educational and helpful in helping you maintain a health and active life. This is not intended to take the place of a medical care or advice.

NQA's Five Treasures Practice Set

This practice set is divided into three sections: 1) Warm-up (for cleansing), 2) Five Treasures Set (collecting and circulating energy), and 3) Closing (storing energy).
(for detailed instructions, see NQA's Five Treasures DVD)

Warm-Up: Shake the Tree

Full body shaking to loosen all the joints and allow the energy to flow. Then shake each leg, hip, knee, calf, and foot individually.

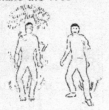

Warm-Up: Twist from the Waist, Swing the Arms

Let your weight shift from side to side simultaneously twisting the waist as soft fists gently tap in front & back of the body.

The Five Treasures

Begin in **calm, centered standing posture**; align body & breath w/calm mind; hands face the dantien (energy spot 2" below navel).

1. Ocean Wave Breathing

Arms round toward center; **inhale**, weight shifts forward as arms move out; **exhale**, weight shifts back as arms return to start position, each time creating a larger wave then gradually return to smaller movement.
Return to calm, centered standing posture.

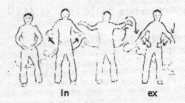

in   ex

2. Draw Up Earth Chi

Bending to scoop earth energy; **inhale** raising arms to stretch overhead; **exhale** moving arms down.
Return to calm, centered standing posture.

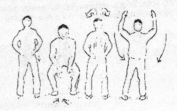

3. Gather in Starlight
One hand behind back at life gate (low back), thumb touching fingertips. **Exhale** as other hand circles forward, then **inhale** bringing energy into each center: (navel, heart, 3rd eye, and crown); reverse gathering movement downward to start position; change sides and repeat.
Return to calm, centered standing position.

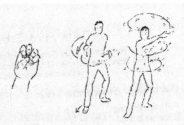

4. Open the Heart
Inhale, reach forward with arms, gather energy into the heart, **exhale**, extend arms out & around to gather again. Reverse direction, **exhale**, as you spread your heart energy out to the world; **inhale** as arms circle back in.
Return to calm, centered standing posture.

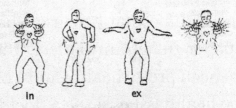

in   ex

5. Draw Down Heaven Chi
Hands turn out to the side, **inhale** as you raise arms overhead connecting with energy, then **exhale**, bringing heaven energy down through the body.
Return to calm, centered standing posture.

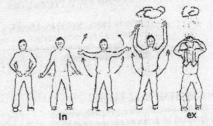

in   ex

Storing and Smoothing the Chi
Begin by using your palm to brush down the inside & outside of the right arm, from shoulder down & off the fingertips. Repeat with left arm. Then brush down the inside & outside & then the front & back, of each leg from hip down off the toes. Use your palms to brush the energy down the front of the chest, from throat to abdomen. Finally, placing your palms over each other, circle the hands/palms over the abdomen in a clockwise direction a few times & then a counter clockwise direction. **Return to calm, centered standing posture.** Feel the energy naturally permeate through your entire body. You may hold this position for a few minutes to complete the practice session.

NATIONAL QIGONG ASSOCIATION*USA
P O BOX 270065
ST. PAUL, MN 55127
www.nqa.org

The purpose of this book is to show you how to get, and stay as healthy as possible without spending more of your hard earned money. It is possible to order DVD's, from NQA to help you with the ideas here, but not necessary. You can do these steps, even if they are not done to perfection, they will help you have a healthy and more pleasant life.

Don't assume that because I have put these words on paper that I am perfect. I am not. Although I have been pretty healthy most of my life, I have had some health issues. I see a doctor on a regular basis and I am on medication as recommended.

I have found over the years, that by doing some of these simple activities each day, my well being has increased. I find I more easily experience optimal health each day. I have lived through the same issues most everyone else has. Difficult relationships, deaths of friends, family & pets. Emotional trauma, financial difficulties, job/career disruption. We all go through these life trials. The more I feel well, the more I am empowered to take control of my life and make better choices.

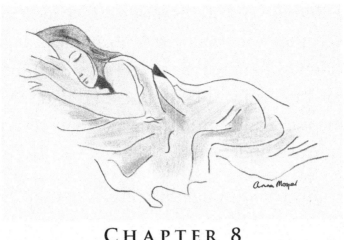

Chapter 8

Sleep, Why We Need It!

Quietly stepping into the room, hearing the soft sounds of a newborn sleeping, breathing in and out almost silently, so innocent and sweet. As you peek into the crib, you may remember your own innocent sleep of childhood. *sigh* Now you would give anything to sleep that sweetly. Sleep is something we all need. We can't function without it. Without sleep we would die. But how many of us just can't get a good night's sleep?. It's not by accident that most good spy thrillers have scenes of sleep deprivation in them. It hits a nerve of truth. We cannot live without sleep.

In the middle part of this past century most people believed that sleep was just a dormant part of our lives. Now we know that sleep plays an important part of our daily functioning and our physical and mental health in many ways that we are just beginning to understand.

We usually pass through five phases of sleep: Stages 1,2,3,4, and REM.(rapid eye movement) sleep. Stage 1, is a very light sleep. We drift off and can be awakened easily. This is the stage we are in when we feel like we are falling or flying and have a "jump". Stage 2, our eye movements slow down and our brain waves become slower. By stages 3 & 4 the brain produces delta waves almost exclusively. It is very difficult to wake someone up in stages 3&4. Some children are so sound asleep that they wet the bed, have nightmares or sleepwalk during this deep sleep. Coming from a large family, my job when we were growing up was to wake the little ones up to go to the bathroom before I went to bed, hoping they would not wet the bed during the night. Most of the time they went to the bathroom in a sleepwalking mode. Their eyes were closed, and they didn't remember getting up to go to the bathroom when they got up in the morning. When we get into REM sleep our breathing becomes more rapid, irregular, and shallow, our eyes jerk rapidly in various directions, and our arm and leg muscles become temporarily paralyzed. Our heart rate increases, our blood pressure rises. When people awaken from REM sleep, they often remember that they have been dreaming. The first REM sleep period usually occurs about 70 to 90 minutes after we fall asleep. Your sleep stages cycle throughout the night. If someone wakes you soon after you fall into REM sleep you may not remember that they woke you up. That's why sometimes you don't remember that your alarm went off, or you took a phone call, someone gave you a message or that you woke up to take your medication You would go right back to sleep and just not remember anything. During REM sleep our bodies heal from whatever stress you may have had during the day. After an injury or surgery you will need more sleep so your body can heal. Sometimes if you are taking antidepressants they repress REM sleep. REM sleep is very important to our well being at all levels. REM sleep also stimulates the brain regions used in learning. I once read a book about a kid who was able to put his book under his pillow and learn his lessons, while he slept.

I though what a wonderful thing! I wouldn't have to study at all! Sadly, it didn't work for me.

If you feel you are not getting enough sleep, see your doctor. If you are a smoker, you may wake up several times during the night. Your body may be having nicotine withdrawals. Many people who have insomnia try to solve the problem with a nightcap. While alcohol may help them fall into a light sleep, it robs them of the necessary REM sleep, and they can be awaken easily. After a while you will understand that your body needs help in balancing its sleep and waking cycles.

The percentage in each stage of sleep is divided up. REM being about 20%, other stages about 30%, and 20% then the cycle repeats itself, over and over until you wake.

The jury is still out as to just how much sleep we each need and how much at what age. You can find lists of age appropriate sleep times everywhere. The most sensible measurement is what works for you in whatever place in life you are at. It stands to reason that an infant will need more sleep then a two year old and a teen needs more than an elder. Depending on what stage of growth or wellness you find yourself in correlates to how much sleep you might need. If you wake up feeling tired, check the most sensible things first. Temperature of the room, comfort of the bed? Too many pets sleeping with you? (We had 3 dogs and a cat! We finally figured it out! They now happily sleep in their own bed!) Constant interruptions. When I worked 3rd shift in nursing, I had to be fierce about my sleeping habits. Once I was down for the count, I couldn't allow anyone to interrupt me. Working swing shift? Try to fix what you can. See a doctor if you need to. Sometimes it could be something as simple as putting on a pair of socks at night to give your feet that extra bit of warmth. Or having a cup of herbal tea before sleep to relax you. I know we are always told to turn off lights and TV so that we can sleep. My husband can't sleep without the TV on! I have learned to fall asleep with it on, as I sleep with him. Once the timer is on, I can relax and will just go to sleep because I know it will shut itself off. If he is working away at night, I just go to sleep in the dark with no problem. I have found that we can adjust.

The more your body is 'growing' or healing the more sleep you may need. A child moving through a rapid growth period may need more sleep then one who has reached a growth plateau, until the next growth spurt. A teen may need more sleep because they are growing bones, muscles and connective tissue, whereas a full grown adult may not need as much. A pregnant woman may need more than a non pregnant one. A person healing from an illness or surgery will need more sleep so that their body can heal. When you have a bad cold, you will require more sleep as you are getting back your health. A healthy older person may not need as much sleep as they did in their 40's or 60's. Getting too little sleep creates a "sleep debt," which is like being overdrawn at the bank. Eventually, your body will demand that the debt be repaid. We don't seem to adapt to getting less sleep than we need; while we may get used to a sleep-depriving schedule, our judgment, reaction time, and other functions are still impaired. Sleep is necessary for our nervous system to work properly. Too little sleep leaves us drowsy and we are not able to concentrate the next day. Lack of sleep also affects our memory and our physical performance. With too little sleep we are not able to do math or figure things out correctly. Without sleep, neurons in our brain may become so depleted in energy or so polluted with by-products of normal cellular activities that they begin to malfunction.

When you are trying to figure the sleep needs of yourself and your family check out the most sensible situation first. If you need help, talk to your doctor.

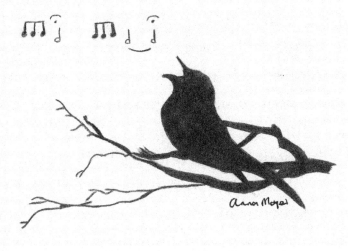

CHAPTER 9

Sounds of Life

Quiet! What do you hear? Did you ever hear the morning sounds rise like cream to the top as your mind comes to life? What is sound? What is a pleasant sound to you? What could a screeching sound be? All different. All individual. All affecting us by what we hear or feel. Sound is vibration. Some believe that we came into being through sound. Our Bible says, "In the beginning there was the Word and the Word was with God and the Word was God." Sound is movement. Some Aboriginal tribes believe we were sung into being. Think of an instrument sounding. Any kind. Think of how a tree or blade of grass makes sound. See the picture in your mind. Hear the sound in your ear, feel the movement of sound against your skin. We are sound. Our body has its own individual sound, its own vibration, unique unto itself. Both sound and light are vibration. If you are in a soundproof room, as you quiet your mind and focus, you can hear the sound of your own body humming, of your blood flowing, heart beating, cells multiplying, your lungs moving air in and out. Did you ever hear the term "listen to the corn grow"? You can. Corn grows so fast that you can actually hear it growing above the ground. All sound from the fine to the gross is vibration. It is part of our life. Vibration is energy. Energy can not be distorted. It always continues. It will change form, but will continue. Anything in the universe that is alive is vibration which is energy in some form. Our plants and pets and us are all energy and will always continue through eternity. If sound and light are both vibration, doesn't it stand to reason that we are also Light? Albert Einstein's theories say this is so.

Biography

Sonja Christiansen is a force to be dealt with, a true overachiever. Her varied areas of accomplishment include practice and credentialing as a licensed massage therapist, small business expert, Karuna Reiki master teacher, and post-secondary level educator. She has held numerous executive level positions in the business world, including a directorship with the American Red Cross, a senior management title with the Women's Business Development Corporation, and a Vice-Presidency with SCORE. She was the founder and managing director of a multilevel company which provided quality speakers & presenters to professional associations providing continuing education credits for rectification in business and healthcare disciplines throughout New England. She has spearheaded a consulting business for many years, providing experts in several areas of healthcare and business management, education, and innovative leadership techniques.

A talented educator, Sonja has taught massage, stress management, and related therapeutic healing techniques at the post-secondary level as well as in smaller venues, and maintained a private practice for over 30 years. She has consulted internationally regarding alternative health practices in such diverse places as China and the Azores.

Her expertise in small business startups and turnarounds has led Ms. Christiansen to provide guidance in the establishment and "course correction" of numerous small businesses, particularly for and by women. Sonja has also served with several Maine gubernatorial advisory groups and task forces with the goal of facilitating and improving small business development. She has been a Delegate with the White House Conference on Small Business, and was a recipient of the US Small Business Administration Advocate Award.

A prolific writer, Ms Christiansen has many publications to her credit which include a collection of anecdotal stories, articles in professional publications such as Developments Magazine, the

Maine Law Review, and Maine Scope, instructional videos and CDs, and of course, books.

When she's not "on the clock", Sonja has devoted time to fundraising to care for stray animals, traveling, rescuing horses (ask her about that one sometime!), tending her garden, and growing young with her man. She speaks parts of a few languages (was born in Germany, actually), is computer cordial, and really has walked on fire.

Cheri Wheeler BSN, RN

BIBLIOGRAPHY

National Institute of Neurological Disorders and Stroke, Internet

National Sleep Foundation, Internet

Holy Bible, King James version

National Qigong Association (with permission)

Nick Ortner, The Taping Solution, Hay House, Inc (with permission)

Home of The Annual World Summits (with permission)

Ann Hill (1979) A Visual Encyclopedia of Unconventional Medicine Trewin Copplestone Publishing Ltd.

John Diamond, MD, (1979) Behavioral Kinesiology, Harper & Row, New York

Hans Jenny, MD., Of Sound Mind & Body, MACROmedia Publishing, Video

Carter-Webber (1994) Body Reflexology, Parentic Hall, New York

List of books, Cd's and classes/ workshops from Healing Focus

Healing Focused Workshops

We offer a variety of full day seminars based on our holistic philosophy, "Your reality flows through your intent." Or a one hour workshop for smaller groups, focused on one topic from this book. Please contact us for descriptions of the wonderful doors you will be able to open into your life

Changing Your Life Through Your Intent

A full day (6 hours) seminar covering each subject in this book. You can host a seminar in your community, school, or church for a few as ten people or as many as 100. Many groups use our training as fund raisers. We will be happy to work with you to help you meet your fund-raising needs.

If you are interested in one on one consultation, workshops/ seminars in your area or books and CDs from Healing Focus please contact us at:

Healing Focus
161177 N. 4334 Rd.

Tuskahoma, OK 74574
918-569-4889
918-415-4424
e mail: infocussonja@yahoo.com
Face Book : FaceBook/Sonja Christiansen
Facebook Web site: Facebook.com/groups/Healingfocus
Facebok E mail: Healingfocus@groups.facebo.com

Books and Cd's available through Healing Focus

Clear Vision, Finding Peace in a Troubled World, ($14.95) Sonja Easy One step at a time learning Meditation. Infinity Publishing.com

Meanderings of an Unkempt Mind, Sonja Christiansen, Woman of Many Hats, Self published. $10.00. A book of chuckles and silliness. just what you need to bring you out of the doldrums. Contact me at Healing Focus or through Face Book.

Healing in the Light, CD, Guided Meditations for Healing and Relaxation. Sonja Christiansen, $10.00 The splendor of Bach though cello, harp and flute, providing a setting for the soft vocal guidance into peace and healing. Order through me or www.KlarityMusic.com

Massage, The Healing Touch - Family Massage DVD $14.95. Sonja Christiansen. Massage is a way to calm and relax loved ones of any age. Learn easy to remember massage movements that you can practice in your own home. Order through me.

I am Your Body, A Healing Focus Program. A great gift for a child or someone young at heart who has undergone the loss of a limb or organ. A personal letter will come from the organ or limb describing it's function and what will happen next. Our letters are uplifting, caring and humorous. Describing how our body will adjust and how the other body parts work together to help heal. Contact us by e mail or phone and we will discuss with you what is needed. The letters are written for young people and will be age appropriate. We will mail any where in the world. Over seas letter s will need extra postage, which we will discus with you. Postage is included for any letters in the US. $10.00.

Just for a laugh, Maine porcupine babies, complete with incubator. Choice of Boy or girl. They will keep someone in your life laughing. "Laughter is the best medicine"! Please contact us.